Healthy life through meals:

Fastidious healthy balance through meal intake for safe eating habits

Chata Lee

DESCRIPTION

Are you sick and tired of enduring strict diets that only last a short while before becoming unsustainable? Are you perplexed by the shifting fads and ongoing debate over what is and isn't healthy? It's time to adopt a straightforward, empirically supported strategy that transcends gimmicks and spares you the stress of rigid macros and meal schedules.

In healthy life through meals, you'll establish a remarkably nourishing eating style that is simple to maintain for life, fine-tune a successful workout routine, put recovery first, and learn potent coping mechanisms. You'll use some cutting-edge methods to achieve amazing body composition breakthroughs when you're ready to level up. You'll learn how to do this while maintaining your energy, focus, and positive attitude

TABLE OF CONTENT

Introduction

Are smoothies a gateway to transmitting a healthier lifestyle?

Chapter 1

Chapter 2

Chapter 3

Chapter 4

INTRODUCTION

Are meals a gateway to transmitting a healthier lifestyle?

Sometimes spending money is necessary to save money. Though Fruits and vegetables that are organic do cost more to buy. It is money well spent if it prevents high medical costs in the future. Considered a good eating habit with a reasonably priced meal, eat more fruits and vegetables, and leave a wonderful life. If you add more protein to the smoothie, you'll have enough fuel and nutrition to last until your next meal. You and your family's tastes may change over time, making the transition to a healthier lifestyle easier. Reduce smoothie's sugar content and change its composition to include healthier ingredients. a way of life that eliminates fast food, processed foods, and sugary drinks is in one favor.

a way of life that moves away from fast food, processed foods, and sugary beverages and toward one in which food serves as medicine. You don't have to eat to live; you can eat to live.

Eating good meals, fruits and vegetables can help you answer the question if meals are the gateway to transmitting a healthier lifestyle

CHAPTER 1

Diagnosing your food intake

Identifying your food intake is an essential component of healthy living as this enables you to track a record of your eating habit. In doing this, you must Determine how long you will keep a food journal. Is it going to last a week, a month, etc.? and to keep track, there are numerous choices such as tablets, apps, calendars, etc.

Your information will be more accurate the more precise and detailed you can be while reporting. It might occur to you that you are omitting entire dietary groups (i.e., vegetables, dairy, on a weekly basis)

Remember to keep track of all the extras, including coffee creamer and sugar, condiments, chocolates from your coworker's candy bowl, beverages, etc. The number of calories in these forgotten delights may astound you. Just 100 more calories could result in an annual excess weight. Additionally, it is simple to eliminate or replace these with healthier alternatives. Monitoring your food consumption will also highlight the things you are already doing well. Continue with these routines to avoid having to start over. Building on your present efforts and making gradual changes to your eating patterns will make you live a healthier life.

Food diagnosing come alongside its importance, which is the basic requirement for human survival. According to the world health organization (WHO), each year 1 in 10 people get ill by eating unsafe food from the safety tips handling developed. These "Five Keys to Safer Food" were created to instruct all customers and food handlers on safe food handling behaviors.

    a. Be hygienic
    b. separate cooked from uncooked
    c. Complete cooking

     d. Maintain food at a safe temperature.

     e. Use raw materials and hygienic water

By seeking the appropriate help and care you need, you can begin to enjoy a life full of freedom from addiction and Unhealthy weight gain, Reduced sex drive, Diabetes, Headaches, Malnutrition, Obesity, Chronic fatigue, and heart disease.

It is important to diagnose your body's intake of food because some foodborne illnesses are contagious or poisonous in nature and are brought on by bacteria, viruses, parasites, or chemical agents that enter the body through contaminated food. Acute poisoning or chronic illnesses like cancer can result from chemical pollution. Many foodborne illnesses have the potential to be fatal or cause permanent disability.

food hazards are mostly prevalent foodborne pathogens that annually infect millions of people, often with severe and fatal consequences, including bacteria like Salmonella, Campylobacter, and enterohaemorrhagic Escherichia coli. The symptom may be fever, headache, nausea, vomiting, abdominal pain, and diarrhea as symptoms.

Some viruses can spread through food consumption. The symptoms of norovirus, a common source of foodborne infections, include nausea, violent vomiting, watery diarrhea, and stomach pain.

parasites, like trematodes found in fish, can only spread through food. Others, including tapeworms like Echinococcus species or Taenia species, can spread to humans through food or close contact with animals.

Prions are distinctive in that they are linked to a particular type of neurodegenerative disease. Prions are infectious agents made of protein.

Listeria infections can cause pregnant women to lose their babies or the death of newborn babies. Despite the relatively low incidence of the disease, listeria infections are among the deadliest foodborne diseases due to the catastrophic and occasionally fatal health implications, especially for infants, children, and the elderly. Unpasteurized dairy products and a variety of ready-to-eat foods contain listeria, which can develop in cold temperatures.

CHAPTER 2

Food Is Your Medicine

Humans have known for a very long time that food has positive health effects. However, many have forgotten that the food they consume is closely related to their health as a result of the creation of chemical medications and tablets. Foods are the best medicine, so we should be careful about how we see and utilize them.

The foods we eat at every meal have a big impact on our health, thus they can also be utilized as medicine because we are what we eat. Good health and a healthy diet go hand in hand. Because food is necessary for human bodies to function properly, any disruption in those functions results from poor eating. For instance, eating meals with a high Glycemic index (the rate at which carbs are digested) can cause a sharp rise in blood sugar as well as a sharp decline, both of which are linked to an increased risk of obesity and cardiovascular disease (Ghartey & Nembhard, 2013)

First, adopting the proper diet and foods to eat can help to improve health and bodily processes. Second, it has long been common practice to use food for health advantages, and scientists are eager to develop meals that help fend off illnesses. The ideas on the health advantages of foods between two generations have certain similarities and changes, which is not surprising. Foods are not really the least, but they are.

Your entire health is significantly influenced by the foods you choose to eat. Numerous nutrients found in food promote a healthy life and shield your body from illness. It's crucial to consume natural healthy foods because there are special components it produces that can't be achieved by taking supplements.

According to research, Dietary choices affect disease risk. While some foods can worsen chronic health issues, others have potent healing and safeguarding properties which is why a lot of individuals assert that food is medicine.

However, a strict diet cannot and shouldn't always take the place of medication. Changing one's food and mode of living can often help prevent, treat, or even cure numerous diseases.

Foods with potent therapeutic qualities

Berries and diets high in berries may offer protection against long-term diseases like cancer.

Herbs like sage, oregano, rosemary, and parsley not only give food a natural flavor but also contain several health-improving elements.

Green tea. The amazing benefits of green tea have been widely investigated by many.

An extensive variety of antioxidants are present in cruciferous vegetables like broccoli and kale. Having a lot of these vegetables may lower your risk of developing heart disease and lengthen your life.

The high concentration of omega-3 fatty acids in fatty fish like salmon, sardines, and other fatty fish guards against heart disease—these fish prevent inflammation. The immune system, heart, and brain all benefit from compounds found in mushrooms, including maitake and rishi.

Spices such as Turmeric, ginger, cinnamon, and other spices are packed with beneficial plant compounds. Based on research, turmeric helps treat arthritis and metabolic syndrome

To generalize it all, Consume fresh fruit and vegetables, whole grains like quinoa and farro, and legumes (beans, chickpeas, lentils). Vegetables have little to no fat and are a fantastic source of protein and healthy carbs. You need 35 grams of dietary fiber every day, and they are a wonderful source of it. Additionally, fiber has been linked to a lower risk of diabetes, obesity, cardiovascular disease, and colon cancer. It is significant to remember that foods like meat, dairy, and eggs lack fiber. Vegetables and fruits both have a lot of phytochemicals (micronutrients that can reduce the risk of cancer). Consume entire fruit instead than fruit juice or fruit that has been canned in syrup.

Fruit and vegetables contain far fewer calories than meat and dairy items. Most of the calories we consume each day come from carbohydrates, which are not inherently bad. Consume the carbs found in whole grains, nuts, legumes, raw fruits, fresh and cooked vegetables, and nuts.

Many American diets are extremely lacking in fiber; only 97 percent of people get the required 31.5 grams per day. Fiber increases the volume of the stool and encourages regular bowel movements. Additionally, fiber has been linked to a lower risk of diabetes, obesity, cardiovascular disease, and colon cancer. It is significant to remember that foods like meat, dairy, and eggs lack fiber. Fiber-rich foods include green leafy vegetables, whole grains, Legumes, and certain fruits.

CHAPTER 3

Eat healthy while living

key things you can do to safeguard your health is to eat a healthy, balanced diet. In fact, lifestyle choices and behaviors like eating a nutritious diet and exercising regularly can prevent up to 80% of early heart disease and stroke.

A nutritious diet can reduce your risk of heart disease and stroke by lowering your blood pressure, managing your weight, and decreasing your cholesterol levels. It can also help you control your blood sugar levels. Eating a variety of healthful foods every day is advised for healthy living. This entails consuming more plant-based diets and avoiding items that have undergone extreme processing.

Eating a lot of fruit and vegetables is one of the most important dietary practices. Fruit and vegetables are rich in nutrients (antioxidants, vitamins, minerals, and fiber) and help you maintain a healthy weight by making you feel satisfied for longer periods of time.

Eating protein-rich food like Legumes, nuts, seeds, tofu, fortified soy beverages, fish, shellfish, eggs, poultry, lean red meats, including wild game, low-fat milk, low-fat yogurts, low-fat kefir, and low-fat and low-sodium cheeses are examples of foods high in protein. To achieve this

> → Protein supports the growth and upkeep of bones, muscles, and skin hence Feed yourself daily protein.

→ Aim to have two servings of fish or more of plant-based foods every week.

Whole grain foods include hulled barley, brown or wild rice, quinoa, oats, and whole grain bread and crackers. The entire grain is used in their preparation. Foods made from whole grains contain fiber, protein, and B vitamins to keep you feeling fuller for longer.

Eat less meat, especially processed meats like canned meat and processed meats like salami, hot dogs, ham, and beef jerky. Processed meats have been identified by the World Health Organization as a Group 1 carcinogen (same category as tobacco smoking). Overall, only a modest amount of your daily caloric intake should come from meat.

Reduce your intake of refined carbs, which can be found in foods like bread, bagels, sweets, sugary cereals, candies, and bagels. Restrict your intake of processed foods, such as fast food, microwaveable meals, pizza, potato chips, and bacon. Your immune system is negatively impacted by sugar and processed meals, which might increase your susceptibility to illness and infection. These foods make the body more inflammatory overall. Whole food plant-based diets, on the other hand, reduce inflammation and promote the growth of beneficial gut flora, which strengthens your immune system.

Reduce your salt intake. Salt consumption should be kept to between 1,500 and 2,300 mg per day, according to the American Heart Association. Salt consumption is linked to cardiovascular disorders such as high blood pressure.

A vital component of maintaining excellent health is exercise. Even if weight loss is not required, it is still crucial. Exercise can enhance cardiovascular fitness, lower the chance of developing diabetes, and regulate blood pressure. You should, at the very least, "huff and puff" for 30 minutes three times a week.

Experts' top five recommendations

    i.   Drink water instead of sugary beverages. Unsweetened, lower-fat milk is another excellent source of fluids. So that you can fill up wherever you are going, keep a reusable water bottle in your handbag or vehicle.

ii. Use whole or little processed foods when preparing most of your meals at home. For variety and to keep things interesting, pick various proteins. You can plan better if you give each day a memorable name. With this meatless meal, try "Meatless Monday."

iii. Take frequent, smaller meals. Consume snacks in between meals at least three times a day. You are more inclined to choose unhealthy foods when you wait too long to eat. Keep quick-to-eat food (like these) in your bag or purse just in case.

iv. Create an eating schedule for the week; this is the secret to quick and simple meal preparation. See here for our purchasing advice.

v. Pick recipes that feature lots of fruit and veggies. At every meal, try to fill half of your plate with fruit and vegetables. Every day, choose colorful fruits and vegetables, especially orange and dark green ones. Fresh produce can be substituted with unsweetened fruits and vegetables that are frozen or canned. Test out this recipe for healthy living.

CHAPTER 4

Smoothies for a balanced diet

Smoothies not only taste delicious but also have a ton of health advantages. Some of the vegetables and fruits' surfaces are reduced when you make a raw smoothie, this makes it easier for your body to absorb some of the nutrients. Smoothies can increase energy and skin tone. This mixture is very strong in the sense that it can provide you with a potent punch of nutrients that will improve the performance of any system.

1. **Celestial cream cheese**
   Ingredient
   1 avocado's flesh
   1 lemon juice,
   5 pitted dates, and
   1   1/2 ounces of seaweed.

Serve after thoroughly blending all the ingredients. Enjoy it with raw crackers, fresh celery, carrots, or another favorite raw snack.

2. **Raspberry coconut smoothie**
   Ingredients
   Low-fat milk, 1/2 cup
   Low-fat coconut-flavored yogurt, 1/2 cup
   Frozen raspberries, 2 cups
   two bananas, peeled and chopped

Blend milk, yogurt with coconut flavor, frozen raspberries, and bananas using an immersion blender. Raspberries and toasted coconut should be added as a garnish.

3. **Green smoothie**
   Ingredient
   250 ml of your preferred milk (unsweetened almond milk is preferable)
   Ground flaxseed, 1 tablespoon
   1 teaspoon maca powder (optional)
   a pinch of cinnamon powder
   smoked 1 Medjool date
   one tiny, ripe banana
   a few handfuls of spinach or Nero
   1-tablespoon almond butter

Add the cinnamon, and ground flaxseed, after pouring the milk into a powerful blender. Blend after adding the remaining ingredients until smooth. Pour into glasses. serve chill

4. **Green mixed smoothie**
   Ingredient
   1/2 pear
   1 1/2 cups baby kale
   CHIA SEED, 1/2 tbsp.
   Apple Cider Vinegar, 1 1/2 tablespoons
   1 cup ice, 1 cup ice, 1 pinch of pink Himalayan salt, and
   1 cup of unsweetened almond milk

combined the above and blend together Until smooth. Ensure the desired consistency is reached, and add more almond milk to taste.

5. Banana smoothie

Ingredient

1 banana

1/2 orange

1/3 cup of Greek yogurt

1/4 cup milk or water

1/2 teaspoons of honey (optional)

Orange and banana should be roughly chopped before being added to a blender. Yogurt and water can be added on top (or milk). Blender should be on and run until smooth and creamy. Taste, and if necessary, correct with honey.

6. Banana raspberry smoothies

ingredient

2 bananas

1 bunch of spinach

1/2 cup of raspberries

1 tablespoon of cashew or almond butter

raw cocoa powder 2 tablespoons

10 tablespoons of unsweetened coconut, hemp, or almond milk

1 scoop of plant-based protein (optional)

Blend all together and served chilled. This smoothie is mainly good for weight loss

7. Cashew and banana smoothie

Ingredient

Cashew nut, 1 tablespoon

½ banana

Full-fat coconut milk in 1/4 cup

2 scoops of Paleo Meal protein powder without dairy

Latte Dynamic Greens, 1 scoop

1 to 2 ice cubes

Using a blender, make a liquid paste from the above list. this has a balance of protein, fat, and carbohydrates that support stable blood sugar levels so that your pancreas can release the hormone that metabolizes calories, glucagon! And because it's so delicious, you can have one every morning without getting tired of it.

8. **Pumpkin Pie smoothie**
Ingredient
¼ banana
1 cup of canned pumpkin
1 cup of coconut or almond milk
Chopped pecans in 2 tablespoons.
1 teaspoon pumpkin pie spice
¾ scoop vanilla Vega protein powder.
½ cup of ice cubes

When you combine pumpkin with protein powder, you'll balance your blood sugar and add the ideal ingredients for a post-workout recovery meal. Pumpkin is a good clean burning carbohydrate.

9. **Pineapple Orange Banana Smoothie**
Ingredient
3 ½ cups of fresh or frozen pineapple chunks,
1 medium banana, peeled, either fresh or frozen
1 large orange(peeled)
1 cup of coconut yogurt
Optional: two teaspoons of vanilla extract.

blend very well until the ingredients are smooth. You can make a smoothie with ice cubes if your fruit is at room temperature.

Spicy Carrot Smoothie

Ingredient

2 cups carrots
1 cup celery
1 tablespoon garlic
Pinch cayenne pepper

¼ teaspoon cinnamon 2
cups water

Blend all of the ingredients until creamy

FOOD HYGIENE

Everyone who works with food either for personal feed or public sales is responsible for ensuring that consumers are protected from contaminated food and the risk of food poisoning, which causes extreme discomfort, absence from work or school and, in some cases, death. People get sick from food poisoning because the food they've eaten has contained bacteria, viruses, or chemicals. It can take from an hour to a few days to develop food poisoning, depending on the cause, and the best way of preventing food poisoning is to use safe food handling practices.

Bacteria are the biggest problem, because they are so common, and are found in soil, on animals, people and even in clothes. In the kitchen, bacteria often come from vegetables and raw meat. Sometimes these bacteria can move from raw ingredients to cooked food, in a process called cross-contamination.
The way that these germs can move includes:

- From hands to food.
- From cutting boards, knives, and other utensils onto food.
- From one food to another, especially from raw to cooked.

Once bacteria are in a food, they can increase their numbers quickly. They just need the right conditions. This means a temperature of between 5°C and 60°C, (sometimes called the danger zone), time and water.

There are six keys to breaking this chain of food poisoning:
1. Someone who is responsible for every aspect of food preparation and sales.
2. Each person handling or preparing the food must know, about and practice safe food handling.
3. Make sure that everything (utensils) used in preparing the food is clean and germ-free.
4. Correct and safe food preparation.
5. Correct and safe food storage.
6. Displaying food safely.

FOOD HYGIENE INVOLVES
   i.   Preventing the spread of infection by people who handle food.
   ii. Ensuring that food preparation areas, equipment and surfaces are clean.
   iii. Protect food from risks of contamination.
   iv. Prevent bacteria from multiplying to levels resulting in ill-health.
   v.   Destroy bacteria in food through adequate cooking or processing.

THE BENEFITS OF FOOD HYGIENE
   1. Return of business through satisfied customers.
   2. Good reputation.
   3. Compliance with the law.
   4. High-quality food and increased shelf life of food.
   5. Good working environment for staff, boosting staff morale and job satisfaction.

THE COST OF POOR HYGIENE

1. Food poisoning outbreaks and sometimes death.
2. Customer complaints.
3. Wastage of goods due to spoilage.
4. Pest infection.
5. Suspension of trading by local health authorities.

APPROACH TO THE PROBLEM

1. Preventing food from being contaminated.
2. Killing bacteria.
3. Preventing bacteria growth and multiplication.

SOURCES OF CONTAMINATION

i. People - (hands, mouth, nose, anus, skin).
ii. Clothes.
iii. Utensils - (dirty utensils, especially those used for raw then cooked foods without adequate cleaning and sanitizing in between, tea towels).
iv. Raw foods - (especially red meat, chicken, seafood, vegetables, water).
v. Flies and pests.
vi. Garbage.

PREVENTION

If we are to adopt the main principles of food hygiene we must adhere to the following practices.

1. Develop and maintain high standards of personal hygiene.
2. Avoid cross-contamination of foods.
3. Establish and maintain correct storage conditions.
4. Clean and sanitize all utensils and equipment used in the handling and preparation of food.
5. Control pests

Food hygiene is concerned with every aspect of food production. The main aim is to promote health. This is the responsibility of everyone in the food industry, from managers to cleaners. All must take great care when it comes to handling and preparing food to prevent unnecessary waste of food, due to spoilage or contamination by moulds, bacteria, physical damage, or vermin.

Most people think that food hygiene is simply common sense, they try to do the right thing and they certainly do not set out to poison anyone. However, when you work in the food industry you must consider several important issues to do with your approach to personal hygiene and kitchen hygiene.

WHERE DOES GOOD HYGIENE BEGIN?

PERSONAL HYGIENE

One of the keys to safe food is good personal hygiene of the people who prepare and serve it. The bacteria that can cause food poisoning can easily transfer from the hands and clothes of the people who handle it to food, so it is important that everyone who handles food has high levels of personal hygiene.

As well as hands, clothes and other body parts, hair and jewellery can contain and spread bacteria to food. Important, too is the health of the people handling food. People with illnesses and those with wounds like cuts and scratches can spread illness through food without knowing it. Good hygiene begins with the attitudes and knowledge of all food service workers. It starts with personal hygiene and caring for yourself. The outward signs are a healthy body and attention to grooming.

PERSONAL HYGIENE AND CONSCIOUS BODY HABITS

As a food service worker, you are responsible for:

1. Practising personal cleanliness:
2. Having a bath or shower daily.
3. Wearing clean undergarments daily.
4. Usinging deodorant but avoid the use of overpowering perfumes.
5. Washing hair regularly.
6. Shaving at least daily, for males without beards.
7. Beards, if worn, should also be washed daily, and kept trimmed.
8. Cleaning teeth frequently to ensure oral hygiene and fresh breath.
9. Keeping fingernails clean. Nail polish not be worn when preparing food.
10. Preparing yourself systematically for work:
11. Brush hair and secure it off the face and in such a way that hair will not contact food or surfaces used for preparing food.
12. Wear clothing which will not cause contamination of foods.
13. Do not smoke in food preparation or serving areas.

14. Wash hands and fingernails thoroughly before commencing work. This is vital because hands are the major contact between the food handler and food.
15. Wear a clean apron.
16. Wear limited jewelry, plain band type rings and plain sleeper style earrings.

PERSONAL HYGIENE AND UNCONSCIOUS BODY HABITS

Following these fundamental rules for good personal hygiene ensures basic standards. However, a food handler also needs to be aware of unconscious body habits and must avoid actions such as scratching or rubbing the head, nose or other body parts, stroking hair/beards, picking pimples, licking fingers when tasting food and the like. Ordinarily, these unconscious body habits do not create problems, but when handling foods for the public, it is not only unprofessional behavior but is potentially dangerous.

THE FOOD HANDLER AS A SOURCE OF HARMFUL BACTERIA

All this focus on the cleanliness of the food handler is because the human body provides a rich environment for micro- organisms to live in. Micro-organisms (eg. Bacteria) are to be found in and on the body. Most of these bacteria are harmless. Many even have an important role to play in maintaining health. (eg. Gut bacteria manufacturing Vitamin K).

However, some are harmful and can cause food poisoning. Apparently healthy people may be carrying pathogenic bacteria without showing any signs of illness.

Everyone must assume that they may be carrying food poisoning bacteria and so take precautions against spreading the disease. It is estimated that 50% of the population carry Staphylococcus Aureus in their mouths/noses. Staph Aureus may also be present in infected cuts and pimples. This food poisoning bacteria may be spread to food by a food handler coughing or sneezing over food, tasting food using fingers or working with an infected cut.

Salmonella and Clostridium perfringens can be present in the intestine of seemingly healthy people. Inadequate washing of hands after going to the toilet may result in fecal material being transferred to the food.

If healthy people are carrying bacteria, then people suffering from nose, throat or chest infections, intestinal upset or skin infections will be shedding bacteria at an even greater rate. If you are sick, you should not handle food. Report any abnormal health conditions. Keep cuts or burns covered with a clean waterproof dressing.

HAND-WASHING

Always wash your hands before handling food. Washing hands is not just a quick wetting under the tap. Adequate washing of hands involves these steps:

i.   Using the hand basin, wet hands with hot water.

ii.   Apply soap. Lather and thoroughly rub over hands, wrists, and fingers. A nail brush is useful.

iii.   Continue washing action for sixty seconds.

iv.   Rinse under warm, running water.

v.   Dry using disposable paper towel.

vi.   Wash your hands again:

After visiting the toilet.

After handling raw food.

After using a tissue, coughing, or sneezing.

After handling garbage.

After changing a nappy.

After handling pets or other animals.

After smoking or touching your hair or other body parts.

SPOILAGE MICRO-ORGANISMS

These micro-organisms alter the appearance, texture, flavor, and odor of food, making the food undesirable to eat. Consumption of spoiled food such as sour milk, does not result in illness or disease.

PATHOGENS

Less than 1% of all micro-organisms are harmful and produce disease. These are referred to as pathogens e.g. viruses, food poisoning bacteria.

VIRUSES

Viruses are the smallest of all micro-organisms. Viruses do not have their own cellular structure, and to become active must enter a living cell. Once a virus enters a host cell, it redirects the activities of that cell towards reproducing itself. Viruses are always pathogenic but are host specific ie. animal cells are only susceptible to animal viruses. Most viral diseases affecting people are transmitted by contact eg measles, mumps, H.I.V., colds, and influenza. However, a few viral infections are transmitted by contaminated food or water. Both Hepatitis A and viral gastro-enteritis are foodborne. Healthy humans produce antibodies, as defense in response to invading viruses. Once exposed to a virus, either through an attack of the disease or artificially through vaccination, immunity is conferred.

BACTERIA

Bacteria are single-cell organisms and their name gives a clue to their shape. Bacteria are important for the aging of meat and in producing foods such as cheese, yoghurt, sour cream, sauerkraut, pickled cucumbers, salami, peperoni, and vinegar. Sometimes bacteria spoil food. Slime and 'off' smells indicate their action. Other bacteria can cause food poisoning e.g. Salmonella. Regardless of their shape, bacteria have the same internal structure and reproduce in the same way. It reproduces by the one cell dividing into two parts. This is called binary fission. Under ideal conditions binary fission can be completed in 15-20 minutes. This means that a single bacteria can multiply to large numbers in a relatively short time. Under ideal conditions, bacterial population can grow from one thousand to over four million in under four hours. Between one and two million bacteria form a serious food poisoning threat.

Under adverse conditions, growth slows down, and many bacteria die. Bacillus and Clostridium have a special way of coping with adverse conditions. They form spores which is a protective means of survival. They go into a dormant state until conditions become favorable again. They are not killed by freezing or boiling while in this 'protective' state. YEASTS

Yeasts are single celled organisms, larger than bacteria. Yeasts reproduce by a process called budding. A small growth appears on the 'mother' cell. As this bulge grows, the mother cell progressively cuts off the new 'daughter' cell. The daughter cell is about half the size of the original cell. It will increase in size until it is ready to 'bud' or reproduce. Yeasts breakdown sugars to produce carbon dioxide and alcohol. This reaction is utilized in the production of alcoholic beverages and bread.

MOULDS

Moulds are usually multicellular but each cell can grow independently. Moulds are often quite visible. They appear in various forms such as powdery blue-green-white patches on lemons, white fluffy patches on tomato paste or blackened areas along the rubber lining on refrigerator doors. Moulds consist of fine thread-like strands called hyphae. The hyphae grow in a mass either across the surface or down through the medium.

UNDESIRABLE EFFECTS OF MOULDS

Many foods such as pumpkin, citrus fruits, zucchini, and bread are susceptible to mould spoilage. Some moulds are pathogenic and can cause infections of the skin e.g. tinea and ringworm. A few moulds produce dangerous toxins. These are of concern in the bulk storage of peanuts and grains. It produces a toxin called aflatoxin. Long term consumption of aflatoxin causes liver cancer.

DESIRABLE APPLICATION OF MOULDS

Moulds are responsible for the flavors and textures of the blue vein cheeses and the surface-ripened cheeses, brie, and camembert. A highly prized sweet dessert wine is made with grapes affected by a particular mould.

Moulds and yeasts are the microscopic members of the fungi group. Larger fungi, mushrooms, and truffles are also used extensively as foods.

Environmentally, moulds are important because of their ability to change complex organic materials into simple substances eg the rotting and decay of dead matter.

Medically, moulds are significant for their antibiotic properties eg. Penicillium mould producing Penicillin.

FACTORS AFFECTING MICROBIAL GROWTH

Micro-organisms form an invisible world around us. They are in the air, on us, on food, equipment, and food preparation surfaces. It would be difficult to find an environment free of micro-organisms.

In some situations, microbial growth will be encouraged e.g. in the making of yoghurt or bread. At other times their presence will be actively discouraged e.g. taking precautions to prevent food poisoning. Either way, to understand how to control micro-organisms, the food worker needs to have some basic knowledge of the conditions required for microbial growth.

There are six factors required for the growth of micro-organisms: 1. Suitable food.

- Suitable water.
- Suitable temperature. 4. Suitable oxygen levels. 5. Suitable pH.
- Time.

SUITABLE FOOD

Microorganisms exhibit a wide variation of nutrient requirements. Some can be sustained on inorganic material. However, the bacteria responsible for food poisoning thrive well in the foods we like to eat, especially those high in protein, high in moisture, and not very acidic.

SUITABLE WATER

- Microorganisms need liquid water for growth and multiplication.

- Dried foods will not support microbial growth providing they are kept dry and tend to be spoiled by yeasts and moulds.
- Most microbes will not grow in high sugar foods.
- Freezing makes water unavailable to micro-organisms
- Food is not the only aspect of a kitchen environment that may supply moisture for microbial growth. Soiled, wet tea-towels, dish cloths, and mops, as well as improperly dried items of small equipment provide suitable breeding grounds for micro-organisms.

SUITABLE TEMPERATURE

Micro-organisms vary in their temperature requirements. Some thrive at low temperatures e.g., Listeria Monocytogenes, while others can live at higher temperatures. Pasteurization will destroy pathogenic bacteria, but not spoilage bacteria in milk.

Bacterial spores can survive boiling. Each micro-organism has an optimum temperature for growth. Below a minimum temperature growth is halted, although the microbe does not necessarily die. Above a maximum temperature the microbe is likely to be destroyed. Bacteria that cause food poisoning grow well at temperature between 4°C and 60°C.

This is called the TEMPERATURE DANGER ZONE. The temperatures in a commercial kitchen fall within the Temperature Danger Zone. Food should not be kept long in the Temperature Danger Zone.

i. Cold foods are to be kept below 4°C.
ii. Hot foods are to be kept above 60°C. This refers to the internal or core temperature of the food.

SUITABLE OXYGEN LEVELS

1. Most microbes are aerobes i.e., need oxygen for respiration.
2. Anaerobes do not use oxygen, and will not grow in the presence of it.
3. A small group of bacteria can grow in either aerobic or anaerobic conditions and are called facultative.
4. All moulds are aerobic, which explains why they grow on the surface of foods.
5. Yeasts are facultative.

SUITABLE PH AND TIME

• Bacteria prefer neutral or slightly acidic environments.
• Moulds and yeasts tolerate quite acidic environments.

Given optimal conditions micro-organisms can reproduce rapidly. Bacteria are the fastest growing microbes. Growth relates to increase in numbers, not size. Micro-organisms need time to multiply enough to cause food poisoning or serious spoilage of food.

FOOD SPOILAGE
Food spoilage may be due to three separate but inter-related factors:
PHYSICAL SPOILAGE
Damage to the protective surface layer of a food item eg. cracked egg shell, dented cans, insect, or rodent damage to packages. This increases the chance of chemical and/or microbial spoilage.

Moisture loss e.g., wilted leafy vegetables, freezer burn on incorrectly packaged frozen goods, staling of bread.
• Moisture gains e.g., staling of biscuits.
• Aroma loss e.g. ground coffee.
• Odor absorption e.g., fruit salad prepared on board used previously for crushing garlic.
• Presence of undesirable objects e.g., stone in a packet of lentils, fish hook in canned fish.
CHEMICAL SPOILAGE
• Chemical contamination e.g., cleaning substances improperly removed from surfaces or equipment.
• Enzyme action e.g., browning or ripening of fruit
• Rancidity of fats and oils.
BACTERIA
Bacteria spoil food rapidly. Foods that support bacterial growth include meats, fish, poultry, milk, and many vegetables. Often the food becomes slimy and develops an unpleasant odor. Bacteria require high levels of moisture, thus do not spoil dry foods. To minimize bacterial growth, keep food surfaces as dry as possible when storing. Foods that are acidic are less susceptible to bacterial spoilage. Also store foods out of the temperature danger zone. Ensure that cold foods are kept cold, and hot foods are kept hot.